Makawee Huaman

NATIVE AMERICAN HERBALISM DISPENSATORY

The Most Complete Herbal Dispensatory.
Recipes, Secrets, And Curiosities Of
Native American Medicinal Plants
To Cure Ailments.
Remedies for your Children Included.

TABLE OF CONTENTS

INTRODUCTION

A newcomer to the world of herbal healing might be overwhelmed by the sheer volume of herbs out there. Over the ages, hundreds if not thousands of plants have been used for all sorts of ailments in traditional medicine and other practices: headaches, colds, skin afflictions, belly aches.

Today, a way of universally navigating that information is lost. Modern medicine and mainstream research are only just beginning to catch up on understanding herbalism, and to navigate this sea of useful botanical information in a way that can be grasped easily by all.

The fact that you are putting all this effort shows a real dedication and commitment to taking matters of your health seriously. There are many prescription drugs out there. However, it doesn't mean that they are the only options available.

For simple ailments, you can always resort to herbal remedies like the ones we will discuss in this book. There is no need to create dependency on prescription drugs. Going herbal is much safer and healthier most of the time. If you are in doubt, always consult your physician first.

Starting out learning herbalism and plant-based home remedies can be difficult, but I hope, and I'm sure, that this book has been an excellent primer for you to continue your journey, get acquainted with the plants, select which ones work best for you, and to empower healing at home.

Even then, there is still controversy about the use of herbs and what they do exactly, which study today strives to clarify. What ancient cultures' herbal practitioners once documented and passed on is only known and kept by a few, and in a fragmented way that lacks the scientific approach.

Even after just scratching the surface of herbalism as a beginner, you realize that learning the art involves knowing all the facets of what each plant does, but where to begin without anything to guide you?

CHAPTER 1: HERBAL DISPENSATORY

Native American tradition

The Native American's healing traditions go back many years when North America's various indigenous groups found that they could heal different medicinal issues by combining roots, herbs, and other naturally occurring plants. But remedies weren't part of the healing process only for Native Americans.

Among these healing practices, herbal remedies play an important part, stretching far off the body's pains and aches, and to the realm of harmony and spirituality.

In general, the herbs and different natural products utilized in remedies are collected from their surroundings, resulting in a further cure range. However, locally unavailable items were often traded over lengthy distances. Medicinal plants and herbs have also been perceived as greatly sacred.

Many different practices have passed on from one generation to another generation orally and in writing never documented, leaving a mystery to many healing remedies. The healers rarely placed their practices or formulas in writing, such as the Cherokee, who created a written language.

They were shocked to see Native Americans recovered from illnesses and injuries they thought fatal after early Europeans came to the U.S. 500 years ago. The herbal remedies of the Indians were much superior in several respects to those familiar to the immigrants. Yet they have no cures for the "civilization diseases," or the diseases of white men, like measles and smallpox, for the Native Americans, who would wipe out many of them during the next some years. These various Native Americans were lost, and knowledge went with healers to the grave. Mostly it has survived until this day, used by both the Native Americans and the non-natives alike, despite losing some of the information. Several modern medicines are focused on herbs and plants that have been utilized by Indians for years. More than two hundred botanicals originally derived from Native Americans are still in use in pharmaceuticals.

Spirituality and Connection:

The difference, both in the past and current, among Native American conventional medicine and healing is the spirituality role in the process of healing. Native Americans claim that there is a connection to everything in nature and that the spirits may promote cause and health illness. Therefore, not just the human physical parts, but their emotional well-being, and harmony of them with their society and the world surrounding them, must be healed. The community also gathered to help a suffering individual with ceremonies, praying, dances, chanting, and herbal remedies.

Today, only science and mechanistic views are focused on modern medicine, although several Native Americans tend to involve the spirit as the inseparable healing aspect.

Healers:

They were often named "Shamans" by European descent people, referred to by their tribes as healers, Medicine Women, or Medicine Men, but Native Americans did not use this term. These healers' primary role was to obtain the world of spirits, especially the "Great Spirit" or "Creator," to better an individual or community.

In addition to being a doctor, a priest was the Medicine Man also. The healers were trained to handle illness in all categories like these, believing that human, natural, or supernatural causes may cause disease. Masks were worn by healers, often horrific and grotesque, to frighten the spirit away that caused the pain or disease. To exorcise the demons, shaking rattles and beating drums when dancing around someone were often used. Medicine Man mixed the right to an exorcism with the usage of animal and plant substances and other practical procedures. Many healers have often used cups or suction tubes, and purification and purging in addition to herbal remedies.

People in medicine have also been born into a family of several generations of people in medicine. Some might have the vision that inspired them to study this. In any scenario, until they became qualified to act alone, anyone who desired to be healers must first spend a long traineeship with some experienced medicine individual.

The healers used the tools made from nature, such as skins, fur shells, bones, crystals, feathers, and roots. Feathers were also used to take the Great Spirit's message, connected to the air and wind. In some cases, the healer can enter a state of trance and obtain the aid of "spirit guides."

In a bundle of medicine, made of hiding or cloth, which was securely tied, healers held their remedies and tools. Different bundle types were used for special purposes, like ceremonies and festivals: the healer's bundles, the tribe's, and bundles. The bundle of medicine contents is sacred, and it is normally forbidden to inquire regarding the personal bundle content. Due to the power they carried to nourish & nurture the group, medicine bundles leading to tribes were often named 'grandmothers.' Medicine pipes, which reflect the ebb & flow of life, are sometimes used in medicine bundles. The smoke exhaled is believed to carry prayers to the spirit. An aspect of individual healing methods is that it's regarded as a personal matter among the patient and the healer. Furthermore, the patient's interests are still valued within his/her cultural values.

Healing Rituals and Ceremonies:

To bring the participants into peace with themselves, their environment, and their tribe, symbolic healing rituals and ceremonies are also conducted. Ceremonies are utilized, but not used for human healing, to assist groups of individuals back to harmony. Some tribes, like the Navajo and Sioux, utilized a medicine wheel, sing, dance, and sacred hoop in rituals that could last for some days, varying widely from tribe to tribe.

Healers could also use painting, dancing, drumming, changing, feathers, and rattles for persons in the rituals of them. Stones (sacred) were often rubbed on the different parts of the human body.

Native Americans also used sweat baths or sweat lodges for purification and purging. It was often thought to remove evils and revitalize the body, used for balancing and healing.

These baths range from just lying in the scorching sun under a blanket to little conical structures covered by branches and hides/blankets. With water, hot stones were covered within the lodge to make the steam bath, and the healer could pray, drum, or sing together for purifying the spirit here.

Sweat lodges have been used for various purposes, often merely to heal a person, sometimes before spiritual ceremonies for larger numbers of people or bringing clarity to an issue. The sage, the best cleansing herb, burnt in certain civilizations till it smoldered and let out smoke clouds. On the skin, it was smudged and was supposed to purify the soul and body, called "sweeping the smoke."

Religious Rights Banning:

The Federal Govt started to ban the religious rights of Native Americans at the beginning of 1882, which influenced their medical methods. Due to their "great hindrance to civilization," the Interior Secretary of the U.S, Henry Teller, requested to end all "Ceremonies and heathenish dances" on reservations. Hiram Price further supported this, Indian Affairs Commissioner, when 1883 report of his stated that there's no reasonable excuse why should an Indian be able to engage in practices that are repugnant to morality and decency, and ensuring better order on reservations requires that such active steps must be taken to avoid and, if necessary, put an end to the effect of demoralizing heathenish rites.

Efforts like these to eliminate Native American traditions result in the Wounded Knee Massacre on 29 December 1890, when attempted to ban by government "Ghost Dance" practice, a movement far-reaching that nonviolent prophesied end to the white American preached and expansion. Goals of Native Americans of living clean, cross-cultural assistance, and honest life. About 150 Native

American men, women, and children were killed when the 7th Cavalry of U.S. was sent to the Lakota Sioux Rosebud and Pine Ridge Reserves to interrupt the participants' dance to be arrested.

While charges were raised against the 7th Calvary participants for killing innocent people, all were found innocent. Two years later, when Thomas J. Morgan, Indian Affairs Commissioner, ordered sentences of around six months in jail for anyone who repeatedly engaged in religious dances/served as men of medicine, more actions were taken to suppress religious practices.

Native Americans focused on their medication for both injuries and illnesses before 1900. At the start 20th century, that began to shift when the IHS (Indian Health Service) opened hospitals and clinics. Although the spiritual harmony of old traditions remained part of the community, many of the Native Americans start to utilize modern medicine, particularly in healing diseases of "white-man" for which no medicine was available to their healers.

After 1978, the Religious Freedom Act of American Indian passage, the ban against Native American spiritual practices remained in place. Unfortunately, much of the healing

CHAPTER 2: USE OF NATIVE HERBS TODAY

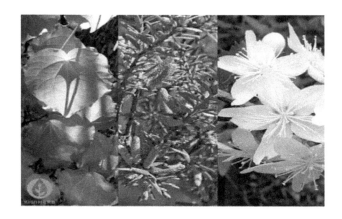

There is a lot about Native American medicine that many people just don't know and certainly don't think about. Of course, Native American medicine may not be as popular as medical alternatives such as Chinese medicine, but these herbs are known to help as well. Of course, with Native American healing and medicine, it was more than just herbs, even if herbs made up such a large part of what Native American medicine was.

Why You Should Use Native American Medicine

Native Americans used leafy vegetables and mashed pumpkins or other materials as poultices. The poultice is placed on the wound or inflammation to relieve pain, increase blood circulation, and draw out pus as in case of abscess wounds.

Herbal medicine has been reintroduced through various ways in the form of alternative medicine. This includes aromatherapy, acupuncture, herbal treatment, and other forms of alternative medicine. Herbal treatment seeks to heal people of common illnesses and other health conditions using herbal remedies, which can be in the form of supplements, tea ingredients, oils, and powdered ingredients. Some clinical herbalists supply Native American herbs that treat health conditions like arthritis, skin problems, asthma, broken bones, hormonal problems, and many other ailments. However, for the herbs to become effective, they have to be taken in the right dosage and combined as recommended. They should also be obtained from controlled sources that ensure quality.

Western medical treatments which use prescription drugs and medical procedures like surgery have been successful in treating various medical conditions. Unfortunately, the side effects are unpleasant. Some people turn to herbal remedies to relieve the side effects. Aromatherapy changes the individual's moods by smelling the scents. This enhances the body, mind, and spirit. Different materials are used, such as oils, leaves, flowers, and candles. The different scents have different effects on the individual. Take, for example, Lavender. It is known to relieve asthma, bronchitis, and other respiratory problems while it brings peace and balance to the individual. Basil stimulates the brain. Some of the aromas used are very refreshing to the body, mind, and spirit.

Alternative medicine has awakened the Native American beliefs and practices by offering help in the form of natural remedies and believes that is now aiming at restoring balance on the physical, mental, emotions, and spirituality as it was intended in the American culture. Alternative medicine based on Native American medicine has become so popular that people are searching for it. People who have chronic ailments are looking for solutions to end their suffering, and Native American medicine is offering hope for these individuals where Western medicine has been unable to help them cope with the chronic ailments and the side effects caused by conservative treatments. Some people are even using these natural herbal remedies to prevent illnesses and diseases by becoming more proactive. Americans natives and non-natives are searching for ways to cure illnesses and diseases with fewer side-effects and less resistance, and addiction with the hope of feeling better, and this lies in Native American medicine, making it gain popularity. Furthermore, some forms of conservative treatments like chemotherapy and radiotherapy are stressful and depressing to the patients and their families. Herbal remedies are not as stressful and depressing because they aim at creating a balance in the individual and harmonizing him or her with the people around him or her and with nature.

Native Americans believed that nature is the most important part of the universe, and we as humans are part of nature. That is why solutions should be sought from nature by restoring balance and harmony with nature. Native Americans believed that the reason why an individual or a community has illnesses and trauma is that there are disturbances in the balance with nature, which should be corrected. The Navajo use healing chants to repair the body, mind, and spirit. They believe that these chants attract a cure for illnesses. They aim at harmonizing the physical, mental, and spiritual to heal various illnesses and physical injuries caused by accidents and trauma.

Today, prescription drugs are expensive, and in fact, most of them are out of reach for many people who cannot afford them. The herbal remedies, which you can find in local food stores and herbal clinics, are known to be less expensive and less toxic than pharmaceutical products. Although alternative healing methods have not been tested as pharmaceutical products have, they have been effective in treating a range of health conditions from complicated diseases like arthritis, cancer, and tumors to common ailments like colds, coughs, headaches, sore throat, and fever. Native American Indians chewed specific plant roots to relieve colds, coughs, sore throats, and headaches, while teas were used for health problems like stomach aches and indigestion. These herbal remedies are still available, and you can prepare them at home for various ailments.

Some over-the-counter OTC drugs and prescription drugs are based on natural ingredients, which are derived from Native American medicinal herbs. There is, therefore, some similarity in both approaches. Both the Native American tribes and the medical society, as we know it has similar approaches to medicine; it is only that they approach it differently. Western medicine uses tested manufactured pharmaceutical products while the natives use herbs, which are in the form of food, teas, and poultices, which are extracted from leaves, roots, sap, fruits or berries, stems, flowers, and other parts of the plant.

Some ingredients in manufactured products are the same as the ones used by the natives. This is because the medical profession depended and still depends to some extent on Native American natural products. Take, for example, Wild Cherry. This is a common ingredient that is found in cough syrups today. In fact, natives have contributed greatly towards health knowledge since many pharmaceutical drugs like aspirin, morphine, quinine, cough syrups, and others contain ingredients that are derived from nature, and many of these ingredients originated from Native American cultures, and these have made a break-through today.

CHAPTER 3: USE OF HERBS FOR AILMENTS

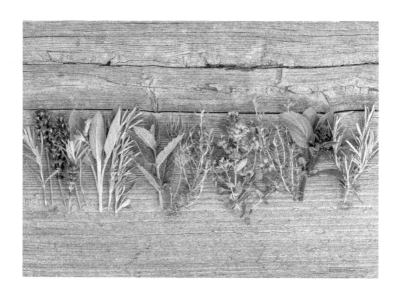

Skin Ailments

Before discussing remedies for bites and stings, you must make sure you seek medical advice for an allergic reaction. If your throat or face starts to swell, go to the hospital to get help. If you get bitten by a venomous animal, also seek medical help. Beyond these warnings, just keep your eyes open for severe reactions to the bite, sting, or rash.

Bites and stings

For bites and stings, you can take fresh lavender leaves or the essential oil, and rub it over the affected area.

You can also apply the juice from one of these herbs: Sweet basil, holy basil, sage, or thyme. Squeeze out the juice, or crush the herbs and collect the juice, and rub it on the affected area. Use only one of these herbs, not a combination of them all.

You can also apply St. John's wort-infused oil to the affected area. St. John's Wort infused oil needs to be cold-processed. Since cold-infused oil takes a while to process, make sure you take the time to make it before you need it. To cold-infuse oil, you should place the 250 g dried herb or 500 g fresh in a large glass jar. Pour in 750 ml good quality olive oil or sunflower oil. Pour the oil over the herbs until they are completely covered. Shake the jar and place it in a sunny spot. Leave for 2–6 weeks, then strain out the herbs, keeping the oil. Store the oil in a dark glass container for up to a year.

Alternatively, you can make a lotion from calendula. To make a lotion, start by making an infusion. Use 2 heaping tablespoons of calendula petals. Add them to a warmed teapot. Pour 150 ml boiling water into the pot. Infuse for 10 minutes before removing the herbs and strainer. When the infusion cools, soak a washcloth in the infusion. Then wring out the washcloth and gently bathe the area.

Finally, you can use the gel from an aloe vera leaf and apply it to the affected area.

If you have nothing else available but have a lemon, then just use the juice of a lemon. Do not dilute it. Use it directly on the affected area.

Rashes

For skin rashes, you can make a lotion of calendula or comfrey (choose one, not both). To make a lotion, start by making an infusion. Use 20 g dried herbs. Add them to a warmed teapot. Pour 500 ml boiling water into the pot. Infuse for 10 minutes before removing the herbs and strainer. When the infusion cools, soak a washcloth in the infusion. Then wring out the washcloth and gently bathe the area. Apply the lotion 2–4 times a day.

If you don't want to make a lotion, you can make an ointment instead, again using either herb. Apply the ointment 2–4 times a day.

If your rash is weeping, apply aloe vera gel to the affected area. Use it 2–4 times a day.

Hives

For hives, drink an infusion of nettle, heartsease, and calendula. To prepare a pot of the infusion, use 5 g of each herb. Add them to a warmed teapot. Pour 750 ml boiling water into the pot. Infuse for 10 minutes, then drink throughout the day. Continue for one week, but if the hives continue after that, you can continue drinking for an additional week.

Another remedy to take is a decoction of dandelion, yellow dock, and burdock. Do not take this remedy if you are pregnant. To make a decoction, place 5 g of each herb's roots, and 750 ml water in a saucepan. Bring to a boil and simmer for 20–30 minutes. It should reduce until there is only 500 ml liquid left. Sieve the mixture, keeping the liquid and discarding the herbs. Drink up to 300 ml a day and continue the remedy for one week.

Chickenpox

The herbal remedies for chickenpox are the same as for cold sores. You can use a tincture of echinacea. Take ½ teaspoon tincture with water 2–3 times a day.

Another remedy is to take an infusion of St. John's wort and drink 150 ml a day. To prepare the infusion, use 1 teaspoon dried or 2 teaspoons fresh herb to 250 ml water. Make the infusion like a tea, with the herbs in a strainer and boiling water poured over. Cover with a lid and infuse for 5–10 minutes before removing the herbs and strainer. Feel free to add sweeteners or honey if you need to. You can store the extra infusion in the fridge for up to 24 hours.

You can also use an infusion of lemon balm. To prepare the infusion, use 1 teaspoon dried or 2 teaspoons fresh herb to 250 ml water. This is one dose. Make the infusion like a tea, with the herbs in a strainer and boiling water poured over. Cover with a lid and infuse for 5–10 minutes before removing the herbs and strainer. Feel free to add sweeteners or honey if you need to. You can drink up to 750 ml a day.

Lemon balm can be an effective lotion. To make a lotion, start by making an infusion. Use 1½ tablespoon fresh lemon balm or 3 teaspoons dried. Add it to a warmed teapot. Pour 150 ml boiling water into the pot. Infuse for 10 minutes before removing the herbs and strainer. When the infusion cools, dab some onto your sores, 3–5 times a day.

To help ease your skin when you have chickenpox, you can take a bath with oats. Place milled oats in the sock end of a stocking or a muslin bag and place it under the tap of a bath. Turn the hot water on and allow the water to run through the oats. Fill the bath and soak for 10 minutes.

Allergies and Asthma

Allergies are usually accompanied by a lot of mucus, irritated eyes, and runny nose. The remedies here can help, but you can also help by changing your diet during allergy season. Foods like milk and other dairy products can increase mucus production, so remove them from your diet to help with the process of healing.

Asthma is often exacerbated by allergies. The remedies for asthma will help for relief, but you should talk to an herbal practitioner or doctor for further treatment.

In case the allergies or asthma get worse after taking a remedy, talk to your doctor. For life-threatening allergies, work with your doctor before taking any remedies. Do not stop taking any steroids or inhalants in exchange for an herbal remedy.

The herbs used for allergies are nettle, elderflower, and echinacea. For asthma, the herbs used are nettle, chamomile, and echinacea.

General Asthma Remedies

Make an infusion of nettle and take 400–600 ml a day for no more than three months at a time. To prepare a pot of the infusion, use 20 g dried herbs or 30 g fresh herbs. Add them to a warmed teapot. Pour 500 ml boiling water into the pot. Infuse for 10 minutes, then pour some out into a cup, but don't exceed the dosage measurements. Feel free to add sweetener or honey if desired. You can store the extra infusion in the fridge for up to 24 hours.

The second general remedy is to make an infusion of nettle and elderflower. To prepare this infusion use, 1 teaspoon dried or 2 teaspoons fresh of each herb to 300 ml water. This is one dose. Make the infusion like a tea, with the herbs in a strainer and boiling water poured over. Cover with a lid and infuse for 5–10 minutes before removing the herbs and strainer. Feel free to add sweetener or honey if desired.

Hay Fever

Make an infusion of elderflower and take 300–450 ml a day. Drink the infusion daily for a few months before and during allergy season. To prepare a pot of the infusion, use 20 g of dried herb, or 30 g fresh herbs. Add them to a warmed teapot. Pour 500 ml boiling water into the pot. Infuse for 10 minutes, then follow the dosage measurements. Feel free to add sweeteners or honey if you need to. You can store the extra infusion in the fridge for up to 24 hours.

Wheezing

Make an infusion of two herbs: thyme and nettle. To prepare a pot of the infusion, use 15 g of each herb. Add them to a warmed teapot. Pour 710 ml boiling water into the pot. Infuse for 10 minutes. Drink it throughout the day. Feel free to add sweeteners or honey if needed.

The second remedy is to make an infusion with German chamomile. To prepare the infusion, use 2 heaping teaspoons chamomile to 150 ml water. This is one dose. Make the infusion like a tea, with the herbs in a strainer and boiling water poured over. Cover with a lid and infuse for 10 minutes. Inhale the steam before removing the herbs and strainer. Drink the infusion, and feel free to add sweetener or honey if you need to.

Asthma from Infections

This remedy has a couple of different options. You can take capsules or a tincture of echinacea. To make the capsule, fill a capsule case with about 500 mg powdered echinacea. Take one capsule three times a day. Alternatively, sprinkle the same amount of powder on food or in water. For the tincture, take ½ teaspoon 1:5 tincture with water 2–3 times a day.

Burns and Sunburn

The remedies here can help with managing minor burns, but you should see a medical professional if a large portion of your skin is burned or if it is infected. For burns beyond sunburn, the best remedy is to keep the wound cool by running cool water over it for at least 20 minutes. Then apply a cool, wet washcloth to the affected area for at least three hours. If the burn is deep or large, seek medical help. The remedies here can also help with burns and sunburns. The plants in this section are aloe vera and calendula, which can be used for both burns and sunburns.

The first remedy is aloe vera gel. To collect the gel, break off a leave from the plant and split it open. Scrape out the gel and apply it to the burned area twice a day.

The second remedy is to apply a lotion of calendula. To make a lotion, start by making an infusion. Use 1 heaping teaspoon of calendula petals. Add them to a warmed teapot. Pour 150 ml boiling water into the pot. Infuse for 10 minutes before removing the petals and strainer. When the infusion cools, soak a washcloth in the infusion. Then wring out the washcloth and gently bathe the area.

Ear, Nose, and Throat

Bronchitis/Chest cold

The herbs that can help you manage your chest cold are thyme, licorice, and two herbs that haven't been discussed yet eucalyptus and elecampane. Eucalyptus leaves are an excellent remedy for getting rid of mucus. It is also a good antiseptic and helps with many respiratory ailments. Elecampane is a root that has been used to help with most chest infections and complaints. Elecampane should not be taken if you are breastfeeding or pregnant. You should also not give eucalyptus to children or infants.

The first remedy is an infusion of thyme. You can have up to 750 ml a day, however, a good option is just to have 100ml three times a day. To prepare a pot of the infusion, use 20 g dried herbs or 30 g fresh herbs. Add them to a warmed teapot. Pour 500 ml boiling water into the pot. Infuse for 10 minutes, then pour some out into a cup, but don't exceed the dosage measurements. You can sweeten the infusion if you want to.

For coughs and bronchitis, you can make a decoction of elecampane. You can add 5g of eucalyptus leaf for acute coughs and bronchitis, and 5 g licorice powder for flavor. Drink about 300 ml of the decoction each day. To make a decoction, place 20 g elecampane root (or 15 g elecampane and 5 g eucalyptus for acute coughs), and 750 ml water in a saucepan. Bring to a boil and simmer for 20–30 minutes. It should reduce until there are only 500 ml of liquid left. Sieve the mixture, keeping the liquid and discarding the herbs. Store any leftover decoction in the fridge for up to 48 hours. Remember, don't take this remedy if you are pregnant.

For an external chest rub (never taken internally), mix 5 drops of thyme essential oil, 5 drops of eucalyptus essential oil, and 2 teaspoons olive oil. Use up to twice a day on your chest and back. Never ingest this mixture, and don't use it if you are pregnant.

Fever

For mild fever, you can make an infusion of yarrow and elderberry; however, this remedy shouldn't be taken if you are pregnant. To prepare the infusion, use ½ teaspoon yarrow and ½ teaspoon elderberry to 100 ml water. This is one dose. Make the infusion like a tea, with the herbs in a strainer and boiling water poured over. Cover with a lid and infuse for 10 minutes before removing the herbs and strainer. Feel free to add sweeteners or honey if you need to. You can drink up to 600 ml a day.

As an alternative remedy, you can take a whole onion, bake it at 400°F for 40 minutes. Mix honey with an equal amount of onion juice. You can take one or two teaspoons of the remedy every hour, but don't exceed eight times a day.

You can also reduce a fever without herbal help by bathing in cool water.

For high fever, you can make an infusion of yarrow, boneset, and cayenne. Boneset is a new herb for this book. You will use the aerial parts of the plant for this remedy. You should not use this remedy if you are pregnant. To prepare the infusion, use 1 teaspoon dried boneset, 1 teaspoon dried yarrow and a pinch of cayenne to 150 ml water. This is one dose. Make the infusion like a tea, with the herbs in a strainer and boiling water poured over. Cover with a lid and infuse for five minutes before removing the herbs and strainer. Feel free to add sweetener, honey, ginger, or cinnamon for flavor if you need to. You can take up to 600 ml of the infusion a day.

Stuffy Nose and Sinus Infections

For congestion issues, the remedy is to inhale the steam of infusions or essential oils.

The first remedy is inhaling the steam of an infusion. To prepare the infusion, use 15 g dried herbs to 750 ml water. Make the infusion like a tea, with the herbs in a strainer and boiling water poured over. Cover with a lid and infuse for 5–10 minutes before removing the herbs and strainer. Then inhale the steam for 10 minutes.

You can also use German chamomile, following the same directions as above. You can also exchange the herbs with 5–10 drops of eucalyptus essential oil or chamomile essential oil and follow the rest of the directions above.

Sore Throat and Laryngitis

All of these remedies will help with sore throats and can also be beneficial to healing laryngitis. You can also simply gargle with warm water and salt for laryngitis.

For a sore throat, you can gargle 20 ml lemon juice. If it's too strong for you, you can dilute it with some water and honey. Alternatively, gargle with 5 teaspoons lemon juice with a pinch of powdered cayenne pepper.

Another remedy is to create an infusion of sage. Do not take this remedy if you are pregnant. To prepare the infusion, use 1 teaspoon dried, or 2 teaspoons fresh herb to 250ml water. This is one dose. Make the infusion like a tea, with the herbs in a strainer and boiling water poured over. Cover with a lid and infuse for 10 minutes before removing the herbs and strainer. Let it cool a little, so it's not going to burn you, then gargle and swallow the infusion. To increase its effectiveness, add 5 ml vinegar and honey.

You can also use a combination of garlic, ginger, and lemon juice. To make this juice, crush a clove of garlic. Wait 10 minutes before you use it. Mix the crushed garlic with a similar amount of grated fresh ginger, the juice from 1 lemon, and 150 ml warm water. Drink up to 450 ml a day. This remedy is also effective for colds.

Gargling a decoction of echinacea root can also be an effective remedy. To make a decoction, place 20 g dried root and 750 ml water in a saucepan. Bring to a boil and simmer for 20–30 minutes. It should reduce until there are only 500 ml of liquid left. Sieve the mixture, keeping the liquid and discarding the roots. Store any leftover decoction in the fridge for up to 48 hours. Gargle 2½ teaspoons three times a day.

Cold

Some of the remedies above can be used to help heal colds and relieve symptoms, especially the remedy with garlic, ginger, and lemon juice from the section on sore throats.

Another remedy is to drink the juice of 1 lemon with ½ teaspoon cinnamon, 1 teaspoon honey, and some warm water.

Using some of your boneset from the fever remedy, you can create an infusion with thyme. To prepare the infusion, use ½ teaspoon dried thyme and ½ teaspoon boneset to 150 ml water. This is one dose. Make the infusion like a tea, with the herbs in a strainer and boiling water poured over. Cover with a lid and infuse for 5–10 minutes before removing the herbs and strainer. Feel free to add sweeteners or honey if you need to. You can drink up to 450–600 ml a day, but don't exceed this dosage.

An infusion of ginger can also be effective. To prepare the infusion, use 3 slices of ginger and infuse in 150 ml water. This is one dose. Make the infusion like a tea, with ginger in a strainer and boiling water poured over. Cover with a lid and infuse for five minutes before removing the herbs and strainer. Feel free to add sweeteners or honey if you need to. You can drink up to 750 ml a day.

For children, you can make an infusion of thyme. To prepare the infusion, use 1 teaspoon thyme to 150 ml water. You can give ⅔–1 cup a day for this remedy. Make the infusion like a tea, with the thyme in a strainer and boiling water poured over. Cover with a lid and infuse for 5–10 minutes before removing the herbs and strainer. Cool enough for your child to drink before giving it to them.

Flu

Again, many of the remedies already discussed in this section can help you with symptoms of the flu. Since flu leads to severe discomfort, these remedies can help with individual symptoms and make you more comfortable.

For muscle aches associated with the flu, make an infusion of thyme, lemon balm, and elderflower. To prepare a pot of the infusion, use 5 g of each herb. Add them to a warmed teapot. Pour 750 ml boiling water into the pot. Infuse for 10 minutes, then pour some out into a cup to drink. Feel free to add sweeteners or honey if you need to. You can drink up to 750 ml a day.

Ear Infections and Earaches

Before we look at earache remedies, it's important to take children with earaches to see a professional before using any of these remedies.

You can use lavender essential oil to help with earaches. Simply use a cotton ball with a couple (2) drops of essential oil and 2 additional drops of carrier oil on it. Put the cotton ball in your ear, not pressed in too far. Leave for an hour, and then remove the cotton ball.

Another remedy is to make a tincture for each of these herbs: Echinacea, thyme, marshmallow, and elderflower. Using equal parts of each tincture (for instance, 3 drops of each tincture), take a teaspoon three times a day diluted in water.

For ear infections, use a large clove of garlic. Crush the garlic and soak it in 1 tablespoon olive oil for 24 hours. Remove the clove, strain the oil, warm it to body temperature and add two drops to a cotton ball. Place the cotton ball in your ear, not pressed in too far. Leave for an hour, and then remove the cotton ball.

Fungal Infections

Fungal infections can be recurrent, depending on your diet and activity level. To help with these remedies, reduce the amount of food you eat with yeast and sugar in them. For each of these remedies, you'll use antiseptic and antifungal herbs like calendula, comfrey, turmeric, garlic, and elderflower. If you have access to tea tree oil, that is also an effective remedy.

Athlete's foot

The first remedy for an athlete's foot is to make a compress of comfrey. To make a poultice, use fresh comfrey if possible, though dry can also work. You should have enough herbs to cover the infected areas of your feet. Place the herb in a pot, and simmer for two minutes without added liquid. Remove from heat, squeeze out any extra liquid, and apply oil to your skin. Then place the hot herb on the affected area and cover it with gauze. Leave on for 1–2 hours every day. Because comfrey is a fast-healing herb, do not use it on broken skin or open wounds.

Alternatively, you can apply ½ of a crushed garlic clove to your feet 2–3 times a day. Garlic is both antifungal and antiseptic, so it will help to clear out the fungus.

Vaginal Yeast Infections

For vaginal yeast infections, you can make a douche or wash with an infusion of calendula. To prepare the infusion, use 1 teaspoon dried or 2 teaspoons fresh calendula petals to 250 ml water. Make the infusion like a tea, with the herbs in a strainer and boiling water poured over. Cover with a lid and infuse for 5–10 minutes before removing the herbs and strainer. Once the infusion has cooled enough, use it to wash the affected area or use it as a douche. Alternatively, you can pour the infusion into a warm bath. Soak for 20 minutes.

You can also make an internal vaginal remedy out of tea tree essential oil. This remedy shouldn't be used if you are pregnant. Mix 2 drops tea tree essential oil with 3 drops olive oil. Once mixed, apply to a tampon and insert it into the vagina. Keep in place for 2–3 hours before removing, and only use it once a day.

Candidiasis

To treat candidiasis, you can make an infusion of thyme, elderflower, and calendula. Drink 300–450 ml of the infusion daily. To prepare a pot of the infusion, use 8 g of each herb. Add them to a warmed teapot. Pour 750 ml boiling water into the pot. Infuse for 10 minutes, then pour some out into a cup, but don't exceed the dosage measurements. You can store the extra infusion in the fridge for up to 24 hours.

Hangover, Headaches, and Migraines

For a hangover, make a decoction of dandelion root. To make a decoction, place 15 g of dried dandelion root and 750 ml water in a saucepan. Bring to a boil and simmer for 20–30 minutes. It should reduce until there are only 500 ml of liquid left. Sieve the mixture, keeping the liquid and discarding the roots. Drink small quantities throughout the day and store any leftover decoction in the fridge for up to 48 hours. To improve the effectiveness of this remedy, make sure you drink plenty of water throughout the day.

For a headache, you can use a temple rub with lavender essential oil. Rub a few drops on your temples.

You can also make an infusion of peppermint to help with headaches. Do not give this remedy to children under the age of five. To prepare the infusion, use 1 teaspoon dried or a small handful of fresh peppermint leaves to 150 ml water. This is one dose. Make the infusion like a tea, with the herbs in a strainer and boiling water poured over. Cover with a lid and infuse for 5–10 minutes before removing the herbs and strainer. Feel free to add sweeteners or honey if you need to. Drink up to 750 ml a day for one week.

For a migraine, make an infusion of rosemary. To prepare the infusion, use 1 teaspoon dried rosemary to 150 ml water. This is one dose. Make the infusion like a tea, with the herbs in a strainer and boiling water poured over. Cover with a lid and infuse for 5–10 minutes before removing the herbs and strainer. Feel free to add sweeteners or honey if you need to. Take up to 600 ml a day.

High Blood Pressure/Hypertension

The herbs used to help remedy mild hypertension are garlic, ginkgo, and ginger. While these herbs can help, so can a change in diet and activity level. Eating a high-fiber diet with low sugar can help to reduce hypertension. If any of these remedies cause you to feel severe chest pain, dizziness, faintness, discolored skin, or tingling, immediately seek medical care from a professional. If you are already taking medication for your high blood pressure, talk to your doctor before taking any herbal remedies.

You can eat 1–2 fresh garlic cloves each day. Remember to wait 10 minutes after crushing the garlic before eating it to get the most out of the herb.

Another option is to take ginkgo tablets. You can also grate 1 teaspoon of fresh ginger into your food or water every day.

Inflammation

Joint Pain and Stiff Joints

For joint pain, use a rub of St. John's wort-infused oil and lavender essential oil. How to infuse the oil will be discussed below. To use this remedy, combine 2½ tablespoons St. John's wort-infused oil with 20–40 drops of lavender essential oil. Massage the mixed oil onto the affected joints.

St. John's wort-infused oil needs to be cold-processed. Since cold-infused oil takes a while to process, make sure you take the time to make it before you need it. To cold-infuse oil, place the 250 g dried herb or 500 g fresh in a large glass jar. Pour in 750 ml good quality olive oil or sunflower oil. Pour the oil over the herbs until they are completely covered. Shake the jar and place it in a sunny spot. Leave for 2–6 weeks, then strain out the herbs, keeping the oil. Store the oil in a dark glass container for up to a year.

A similar remedy is to make a rub of comfrey-infused oil and lavender essential oil. Follow the same process for the previous remedy. Comfrey-infused oil needs to be hot processed. To hot-infuse oil, place the 250 g dried herb, or 500 g fresh in a large glass bowl over boiling water in a saucepan (like a double boiler, but with a glass container on top). Pour in 750 ml good quality olive oil or sunflower oil. Stir the herb and oil mixture and simmer gently for 2–3 hours. Strain out the herbs, keeping the oil. Make sure you press out all of the oil. Store the oil in a dark glass container for up to a year.

Pink Eye

For pink eye, you're going to use two herbs that haven't been discussed yet. Eyebright and cornflower can make an infusion for healing pink eye. To prepare the infusion, use 1 teaspoon dried of either herb, not both together, to 250 ml water. This is one dose. Make the infusion like a tea, with the herbs in a strainer and boiling water poured over. Cover with a lid and infuse for 5–10 minutes before removing the herbs and strainer. Let it cool until the infusion is warm, not hot, and then using a small cup, bathe your eyes. Don't use it more than twice a day.

Arthritis

For arthritis, the first remedy is a change in diet. If you remove acidic foods like tomatoes and oranges (but no lemon), it can help with inflammation.

An herbal remedy for arthritis is to drink lemon juice. Using one lemon, squeeze out the juice and drink it either plain or diluted with water. Drink it every morning.

Alternatively, using three herbs we haven't discussed yet, you can use a decoction of devil's claw tuber, white willow bark, and celery seeds. Do not take this if you are pregnant, taking anticoagulants, have gallstones or peptic ulcers, or are allergic to aspirin. Despite all of the warnings, these three herbs are incredibly useful for treating arthritis. To make a decoction, place 8 g of each herb and 750 ml water in a saucepan. Bring to a boil and simmer for 20–30 minutes. It should reduce until there are only 500 ml of liquid left. Sieve the mixture, keeping the liquid and discarding the herbs. This is four doses. Take 2–3 doses per day. Store any leftover decoction in the fridge for up to 48 hours.

Mouth Ailments

Cold Sores and Herpes

For cold sores, you can use a tincture of echinacea. Take ½ teaspoon tincture with water 2–3 times a day.

Another remedy is to take an infusion of St. John's wort and drink 150 ml a day. To prepare the infusion, use 1 teaspoon dried, or 2 teaspoons fresh herb to 250 ml water. Make the infusion like a tea, with the herbs in a strainer and boiling water poured over. Cover with a lid and infuse for 5–10 minutes before removing the herbs and strainer. Feel free to add sweeteners or honey if you need to. You can store the extra infusion in the fridge for up to 24 hours.

Alternatively, apply fresh ginger, garlic, or lemon juice to unopened cold sores. Use this remedy up to six times a day.

You can also use an infusion of lemon balm. To prepare the infusion, use 1 teaspoon dried, or 2 teaspoons fresh herb to 250 ml water. This is one dose. Make the infusion like a tea, with the herbs in a strainer and boiling water poured over. Cover with a lid and infuse for 5–10 minutes before removing the herbs and strainer. Feel free to add sweeteners or honey if you need to. You can drink up to 750 ml a day.

Lemon balm can be an effective lotion. To make a lotion, start by making an infusion. Use 1½ tablespoons fresh lemon balm or 3 teaspoons dried. Add them to a warmed teapot. Pour 150 ml boiling water into the pot. Infuse for 10 minutes before removing the herbs and strainer. When the infusion cools, dab onto your cold sores 3–5 times a day.

Canker Sores

For canker sores, make an infusion of sage and use it as a mouthwash. To prepare the infusion, use 1 teaspoon dried, or 2 teaspoons fresh herb to 250 ml water. Make the infusion like a tea, with the herbs in a strainer and boiling water poured over. Cover with a lid and infuse for 5–10 minutes before removing the herbs and strainer. Once it's cool enough, use the infusion as a mouthwash.

Teething

For children who are teething, you can make an infusion of German chamomile. To prepare the infusion, use 1 teaspoon dried chamomile flowers to 150 ml water. This is one dose. Make the infusion like a tea, with the herbs in a strainer and boiling water poured over. Cover with a lid and infuse for 5–10 minutes before removing the herbs and strainer. Once it's cool enough, children can take up to 450 ml a day. Alternatively, you can take this infusion and mix with a bit of slippery elm powder and rub it on the gums.

Toothache

For a toothache, chew a whole clove (Eugenia caryophyllata) 2–3 times a day for up to three days. Alternatively, use 1–2 drops clove essential oil and rub it onto the affected tooth.

Gingivitis

To combat gingivitis, take the gel from an aloe vera plant and make it into juice. Use it as a mouthwash 2–3 times a day.

Alternatively, you can create an infusion of sage and use it as a mouthwash. To prepare the infusion, use 1 teaspoon dried, or 2 tablespoons fresh herb to 500 ml water. Make the infusion like a tea, with the herbs in a strainer and boiling water poured over. Cover with a lid and infuse for 5–10 minutes before removing the herbs and strainer. Once it is cool, use it as a mouthwash 2–3 times a day.

Pain Management

Muscle Soreness

For muscle soreness, you can put an infusion of thyme or rosemary into a bath and soak for 20 minutes. To prepare a pot of the infusion, use 25 g rosemary or thyme (not both). Add them to a warmed teapot. Pour 750 ml boiling water into the pot. Infuse for 10 minutes, strain, and then pour it all into a warm bath. Soak for 20 minutes.

Cramps

For cramps, you can use a tincture of cramp bark, an herb that is used as a muscle relaxant. For the remedy, take a mix of 1 teaspoon cramp bark tincture and water. Take this remedy up to three times a day. You can also take the same tincture and rub it into the cramping area.

CHAPTER 4: MEDICINAL REMEDIES FOR YOUR CHILDREN

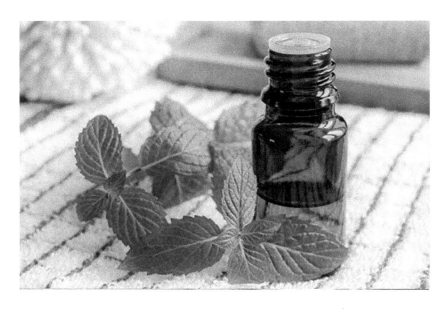

Here is a list of essential herbs and the age groups most appropriate for them. Starting with a newborn, you can add the essential oils to the list for the other age groups, but you cannot add them in regression.

2-12 months

- *Newborn* Dill (Anethum graveolens)

This essential oil is good for colic, flatulence, and indigestion.

- Lavender (Lavandula angustufolia)

Lavender is the most versatile of the essential oils. You can combine it with virtually every other oil in the market; you can use undiluted sparingly without side effects, and it can be used for a multitude of health reasons:

Dermatitis, earache, eczema, psoriasis, sunburn muscle aches, asthma, bronchitis, whooping cough, colic, flatulence, nausea, flu, insomnia, headache, nervous tension, and dry scalp. That is just the shortlist.

- Roman Chamomile (Chamaemelum nobile)

Highly recommended for sensitive skin, this essential oil has a long list of benefits as well:

Acne, allergies, dermatitis, earache, eczema, insect bites, rashes, nausea, indigestion, colic, insomnia, and nervous tension to name a few.

- Yarrow (Achillea millefolium)

This essential oil is not as famous as the two above it, but it does come in handy for helping with acne, the treatment of burns, eczema, rashes, lessening scars, toning the skin, cramps, flatulence, indigestion, colds, breaking fevers, flu, insomnia, and is often added to hair rinses.

Geranium (Pelargonium graveolens)

This floral oil has been used in the treatment of bruises, burns, congested skin, dermatitis, eczema, oily complexions, tonsillitis, sore throats, and nervous tension. *Can cause dermatitis in highly sensitive skin.*

Tangerine/Mandarin (Citrus reticulata)

This essential oil is labeled as one or the other in most natural health stores and online. This is why you should include the Latin name of the oil. This oil is known to help with congested and oily skin, lightening of scars, a skin toner, intestinal problems, digestive problems, insomnia, nervous tension, and restlessness.

Eucalyptus (Eucalyptus globulus)

Well known for being used in vaporizers and other diffusion devices, eucalyptus has been used to open nasal passages and congested chests. It can also help treat insect bites, skin infections, ease muscular aches and pains, sprains, and throat infections. It is also effective in treating bronchitis, sinusitis, colds, flu, and measles.

12 Months-5 Years

Palmarosa (Cymnopogon martinii)

This essential oil has been known to help with acne, dermatitis, minor skin infections, scarring, facials, oily skin, dry skin, intestinal infections.

5 Years - 12 Years

Clary Sage (Salvia sclarea)

This is another strong essential oil, but it's good for use in this age rage. Since it is a little more potent than the ones before it, I would not recommend making it the mainstay of a blend. Two to three drops should be enough for a tablespoon. This oil is good to help with acne, dandruff, oily skin and hair, muscular aches and pains, intestinal cramps, and flatulence.

Nutmeg (Myristica fragrans)

This aromatic oil is used to help treat muscular aches and pains, flatulence, indigestion, nausea, and bacterial infections.

Warning not to use the remedies in the book to treat illnesses without proper medical support

Make Sure to See a Specialist:

You must be seeing someone who can help you through the process of using Herbal medicine properly, especially if you actually wish to use Ayurvedic medicine. You can usually find a specialist in your area, and they will help you actually to get through the process. Though, it will also be important that you talk to your normal doctor as well.

Your doctor may be able to actually give you a referral to help you get to an accredited specialist that will help you through the process. Your doctor can also help you to determine if you can actually use Indian medicinal herbs without interacting with any of the modern medicine that you are taking, including over-the-counter medication. This means that you will need to make a list of the over-the-counter medication that you are currently taking.

Remember that Your Insurance May Cover It:

Not every insurance will cover Indian medicine, such as Ayurvedic medicine, but some insurances will. This is because some insurances will cover alternative medicines, which can include Indian medicine. Ayurvedic medicine is becoming more and more popular in the U.S., allowing for more insurances to cover it. You can also check out what it would cost you to go to a specialist out of pocket, and you can discuss with your doctor if they feel they are capable of leading you through some of the most basic Indian medicinal practices to make sure that you are safe while using Herbal medicine as an alternative.

Read Up on the Particular Herb or Herbal medicines a Whole:

It is important to have knowledge on your side when you wish to start any alternative medicine, and that does include Herbal medicines well. This means that you need to read up on any particular herb that you are planning to use, and you need to know more about this than just the ailment that it can treat. It can also be important to know where it is native, as it will help you to get a better-quality product when it comes to buying the herb. You should also understand a little more about Herbal medicines as a whole since it will help you to understand a little more about how the herbs and treatments are meant to be used to get the most out of them.

Remember that Herbal medicine isn't for Everyone:

One of the most important things to remember is that Herbal medicine isn't actually for everyone. Some ailments really do need modern medicine to help them, such as cancer. Sometimes, Indian medicine, like any other alternative medicine, will only treat symptoms. This sometimes isn't worth it for some people. This means that Herbal medicine isn't for everyone, and you need to make sure that you feel it is the right fit for you before you try it out.

CHAPTER 5: RECIPES

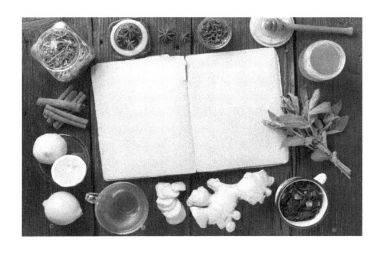

1. *Vitamin C Pills*

Used for:

Vitamin C tablets are useful for helping to boost the immune system, and fight off colds and flu-like symptoms.

Ingredients:

- *1 tablespoon rose hip powder* (the fruit of a rose plant, which has a high Vitamin C content)

- *1 tablespoon amla powder (*an Indian gooseberry, which has strong antibacterial properties*)*
- *1 tablespoon acerola powder (*a Barbados cherry, which is great for stomach discomfort*)*
- Honey
- *Orange peel powder (optional) (*orange is a citrus fruit, and its peel is often used for flavor*)*

Directions:

1. Blend the powdered herbs, smoothing out any clumped powder. Pour a few droplets of slightly warmed honey into the powdered mix. Stir, add a few more droplets and stir again. Mix until the combination holds together without being too sticky or moist.

2. Shape the mix into pea-size balls. Roll these around in the orange powder if you've selected to use it. The mixture should make 45 balls. Store these in an air-tight container to give them an extended shelf life. Take 1-3 daily.

2. Hyssop Oxymel

Used for:

Great for colds, flu, and bronchitis.

Ingredients:

- *Hyssop, fresh or dried (*an herbaceous plant with antiseptic and expectorant properties*)*
- Honey
- *Apple Cider Vinegar (*vinegar made from cider that is great for weight loss and heart health*)*

Directions:

1. Fill a jar lightly with chopped fresh hyssop. (Only half fill it if you're using dried hyssop).
2. Then, fill the jar with honey just 1/3 of the way, and top it off with the apple cider vinegar.
3. Let it sit for 2-4 weeks in the sealed jar before straining.

For a congested cough, you can take 1-2 teaspoons of this remedy every hour. Keep the hyssop oxymel in the fridge for better preservation.

For more information, watch the following video: DIY Herbal Infusions.

3. Oat straw Infusion

Used For:

This oat straw infusion is great for its calming, stress-relieving effect.

Ingredients:

- *2 oz of the oat straw herb (*comes from Avena sativa, which has long-lasting energy effects*)*
- Boiling water

Directions:

1. Put oat straw into a 1-quart jar, then pour boiling water over the herb. Cap it with an air-tight lid.
2. Allow the mix to rest for 4-6 hours, which will infuse the minerals throughout the solution.
3. Strain it. If you choose to, you can add a little extra to your mixture once it's made; lavender, lemon verbena, rosemary, etc.

Oat straw can be used as a base for juices, lemonades, and frozen concentrates. You can use it to create ice cubes or ice pops if you want a variation.

4. *Lemon Balm Home Remedy*

Used For:

Perfect for cold sore sufferers as a natural way to help prevent and get rid of the virus's effects.

Ingredients:

- 2 teaspoons lemon balm, dried (alternate: 2 lemon balm tea bags)
- 1 cup water, boiled

Directions:

1. Boil water, then steep lemon balm for 10-15 minutes. Strain.
2. Use a soaked cotton ball to apply the mixture directly on the cold sore. Use at least 4 times daily. Alternately, try consuming a couple of cups of tea per day to help expel the virus.

5. *Meadowsweet Elixir*

Used For:

This is a fantastic home remedy for pain relief.

Ingredients:

- *100 g meadowsweet flowers* (a European flower that is known as 'the stomach corrector')
- *40 ml 50% vodka* (a distilled alcoholic drink that consists primarily of water and ethanol)
- *100 ml glycerin* (a sugar-alcohol compound often used in elixirs and skincare products)

Directions:

1. Place the meadowsweet flowers in a jar, and then add the vodka and glycerin. Shake well and let it macerate for 4-6 weeks.
2. Check the mixture often, as sometimes the flowers will soak up the alcohol and glycerin so that the liquid no longer covers the herb. In this case, you

either need to use a stone to weigh them down or add more alcohol.

3. After the 4-6 weeks, you need to strain the mixture to be ready for use.

6. Elderberry Gummy Bears

Used For:

These Vitamin C treats are good for an immune system-boosting treat that looks after your well-being.

Ingredients:

- 50 g elderberries, dried
- 30 g rosehips, dried
- 15 g cinnamon chips
- 7 g licorice root
- *0.5 g pepper, freshly ground (*a flowering vine, which is often used for seasoning*)*
- 3 cups apple cider
- *3 tablespoons gelatin (*derived from collagen and used as a gelling agent in food*)*

Directions:

1. Place all of the ingredients (minus the gelatin) into a medium-size saucepan. Bring the mixture to

simmer and continue to simmer for 20 minutes. Strain, squeeze well to extract the juice.

2. Measure 2 cups juice (you can add more apple cider to make the mixture fill 2 cups). Put 1/2 cup into the fridge, then after it's chilled, dust the gelatin on top of it. Allow this to sit for one minute.

3. Bring the rest of the mixture to a simmer. Combine the hot juice with the cooled gelatin mixture. Stir quickly with a whisk. Continue to mix until the gelatin is completely dissolved. If you want to sweeten this up more, add sugar or honey.

4. Pour this mixture into molds and refrigerate. Once they have hardened, they are ready to eat. Eat 1-3 gummies per day, and keep them stored in a sealed container in the fridge.

7. *Bitter Digestive Pastilles*

Used For:

For sufferers of bitter deficiency syndrome or for promoting a healthy digestive system.

Ingredients:

- *1/2 teaspoon angelica root powder (*a European herb used for gastrointestinal tract disorders*)*
- *1/4 teaspoon gentian root powder (*grows in Alpine habitats and treats digestive issues*)*
- 1/4 teaspoon coriander powder (*great for promoting healthy digestion*)
- 1/4 teaspoon orange peel powder
- 1/8 teaspoon black pepper, freshly ground
- 1 teaspoon natural sweetener (for example, honey)
- *1 teaspoon powdered fennel seed (*contains anethole and polymers, which help stomach issues*)*
- 1/8 teaspoon fine sea salt (*primarily used for flavor)*

Directions:

1. Mix all of the powdered herbs, except the fennel seed powder and the sea salt, in a bowl. Then, gently heat up the honey in a small saucepan just until it is thinner and more syrupy. Little by little, pour the honey into the powdered herbal mixture, constantly stirring until it can be molded into pea-shaped balls.

2. Roll these balls into the fennel seed powder and sea salt to create a coating. Store these in an airtight container and enjoy one 15 minutes before each meal.

For more information, watch the following video: Herbal Remedies You Make at Home.

8. Echinacea Remedy

Used For:

This remedy is perfect for canker sores.

Ingredients:

- 2 tablespoons sage tincture
- 2 tablespoons echinacea tincture
- 2 tablespoons lemon balm tincture

Directions:

Combine the three tinctures in a dropper bottle. Use one dropper full of the mixture to swish around your mouth 2-3 times daily.

9. *Homemade Mouthwash*

Used For:

This mixture is a great way to keep your mouth fresh and healthy.

Ingredients:

- 1/2-ounce echinacea tincture
- 1/4-ounce Oregon grape root tincture
- *1/8-ounce plantain tincture* (generally used for cooking due to its sweet taste)
- 1/8-ounce propolis tincture

Directions:

Mix all of the tinctures together in a bottle. Add 30-60 drops to 1 mouthful of water. Swish it in your mouth for 20-30 seconds.

10. Chamomile Remedy

Used For:

The remedy is brilliant for clearing a stuffy nose. Repeat as needed.

Ingredients:

- 2 handfuls chamomile flowers, dried
- 10 chamomile tea bags (*a relaxing, rejuvenating herb*)
- Boiled water

Directions:

Boil 2 quarts of water, then turn off the heat and put in the dried chamomile flowers. Cover the pot and leave for 15 minutes before placing it on a heating pad. Place a towel over your head as you breathe in the steam by leaning over the pot; this will help unblock your sinuses.

11. Rosemary-Infused Oil

Used for:

Hair growth, mental clarity, pain reduction, the common cold.

You can use this infused oil for a hair mask, for cooking, and in balms and salves.

Ingredients:

- Rosemary leaves
- Carrier oil (like olive oil)

Tools:

- Quart jar
- Cheesecloth
- Glass bottles

Directions:

*This method doesn't have specific measurements; it's okay to eyeball it.

1. Rinse your rosemary, making sure to dry completely. Put the herbs in a quart jar with 1-3 inches of space on top. For a multipurpose infusion, olive oil is a great choice. Fill the jar with olive oil, covering the herbs by at least 1 inch. Close the lid tightly and shake well.

2. Jar in a sunny windowsill and let it infuse for *at least* 3 weeks, shaking once or twice a day. We've seen formulas that let the rosemary infuse for up to a month. If the sun is really hot, you can cover the jar with a paper bag. When infusion time has passed, strain the oil through a cheesecloth into a cup or bowl. With a funnel, pour into clean glass bottles. On the label, write "Rosemary oil with olive oil" and the date. Store in a dry, cool, dark place for up to a year.

Directions for dried rosemary method:

*Oil made using this method should not be ingested.

An oil infusion with ground dried herbs and alcohol creates a very potent mixture. You will need to measure out the ingredients. You'll need:

- 1-ounce rosemary, dried
- ½-ounce alcohol
- 8-ounces oil

1. Grind your rosemary into a coarse powder. Don't pulverize it completely into dust, or it will be hard to strain. Move ground herbs into a clean jar. Pour in ½-ounce alcohol. Close the lid tightly and shake well. Wait for 24 hours.

2. Pour the herb/alcohol mixture into a blender or food processor. Start with about 8-ounces of your oil. You want enough oil so that the herbs move around well when they're being blended. Blend for about 5 minutes.

3. Strain oil through a cheesecloth-lined, fine-mesh strainer into a bowl. Squeeze out the cheesecloth to get as much oil as possible. Funnel into glass dropper bottles and labels. Store in a cool, dark, dry

place for up to a year. For increased shelf stability, add a drop of vitamin E extract.

12. Calendula Salve

Used for:

Eases skin irritation, dried skin, eczema, wound healing.

Calendula has antifungal, antibacterial, and anti-inflammatory properties. A salve made with this herb is great for chapped lips, dry hands, cuts, scrapes, and bruises.

Ingredients to make the calendula oil:

- Calendula flowers, dried
- Coconut oil
- Vitamin E oil

Ingredients to make the salve:

- 4-ounces calendula-infused oil
- ½-ounces chopped beeswax

Directions for the oil:

1. If your coconut oil is solid, warm it very gently until it turns to a liquid.
2. Put dried calendula flowers in a glass jar (leaving about ¼ of it empty) and fill with oil, so the flowers are covered.
3. Label your jar. Put the jar in a sunny windowsill and gently shake every 2-3 days. After at least 3 weeks, the oil will be thoroughly infused. The longer you infuse, the more potent the oil will be. Add a drop of vitamin E oil for longer shelf stability.

Directions for the salve:

1. In a double boiler, add your infused oil and beeswax.
2. Heat and stir, so the beeswax melts and mixes in smoothly with the oil. Remove from the heat and funnel into a glass jar or tin. Let the salve cool before closing the lid.

3. Label the container, remember also to write down the date. Store in a cool, dry, and dark place. When using the salve, don't scoop out with your finger, as this increases the risk of contamination. Use a swab. When stored properly, this salve can last up to 3 years.

13. Tulsi-Chamomile Tea

Used for:

Decreases cholesterol levels, eases stress, lowers blood sugar, and helps cold symptoms.

Tulsi, also known as holy basil, is packed with antioxidants. Chamomile also has many medicinal benefits, including anti-inflammatory compounds. Together, they make a tea that can help ease cold symptoms, stress, and improve your heart health.

Ingredients for fresh tea (makes five 1-cup servings):

- 5 cups water
- Handful holy basil leaves, fresh (or 1 ½ tablespoon holy basil, dried)
- 2 tablespoons chamomile flowers, fresh (or 1 tablespoon chamomile flowers, dried)
- Raw honey to taste

Directions:

Steep fresh leaves and flowers in the hot water for 5-10 minutes. Strain and sweeten to taste. You can also drink this tea cold by serving it with ice. If you're using dry leaves and flowers, you use less because dry herbs have a more intense flavor.

14. Aloe Burn Relief

Used for:

Eases sunburn pain, mild burns, psoriasis.

Aloe is a very common ingredient in sunburn ointments. In its natural state, it helps heal and moisturize the skin. It helps with just about any skin issue involving redness and itchiness.

Ingredients:

- Piece of aloe vera leaf

Directions:

This is probably the easiest remedy you'll come across. If you've never used aloe before, always test it in a small area of your skin first, so you're sure you aren't allergic to it.

1. Simply cut the tip off one of the leaves, making sure to cut at an angle (just not straight across), and leaving at least some of the leaves left. With a knife,

carefully split the leaf in half, revealing the gel. Rub gel directly on your burn. That's it!

15. Cleansing Aloe Water

Used for:

Detoxing, constipation relief, heartburn relief.

This aloe water can help with stomach issues, like constipation.

People also drink aloe water to boost their energy and immunity. If you haven't eaten aloe before, we recommend talking to a professional first.

Only ingest only a small amount at a time as aloe can have laxative effects.

Ingredients:

- ½-teaspoon or 1 tablespoon aloe gel
- 1 cup water

Directions:

1. Scrape out gel from a fresh-cut leaf into a blender or food processor. If you have never ingested aloe before, start with just ½ teaspoon.
2. Blend with water and drink!

To make the beverage tastier, you can add other ingredients like 100% fruit juice, cucumber, parsley, or raw honey.

16. Elderberry Syrup

Used for:

Cold and flu.

Elderberry syrup is one of the most popular herbal remedies. Homemade concoctions come with risks since the berries contain components that *must* be deactivated through heat. If they aren't deactivated, the syrup can actually make you sicker. Elderberry syrup should be avoided in long-term, large doses if you have an autoimmune condition. Talk to your doctor before use. The following formula comes from the Franklin School of Integrative Health Science (Hawkins, Hires, Dunne, & Baker. (2019) The Proper Way to Make Elderberry Syrup.

Ingredients:

- 100 grams dried elderberries
- 1-2 quarts cold, distilled water
- 1 ½ cup raw honey

Directions:

Combine water and berries in a large stockpot. Soak for 30-60 minutes. Move to a burner on medium heat and slowly bring to a boil. When you've got a rolling boil, reduce the heat to a simmer. Cook for 30-45 minutes, stirring frequently and leaving the lid off the pot. Potentially dangerous toxins are removed during this cooking process. When time is up, remove the pot from the heat and cool to room temperature.

Strain mixture and measure. It should be about 2 cups. If it's less, add water until you get 2 cups. If you have more than 2 cups, boil the mixture down. For dosing purposes, it needs to be very close to 2 cups. Mix with honey. Return the pot to the stove and bring to a boil again. Cook for 10-30 minutes until the mixture is thick and syrupy. Measure how much you have in tablespoons and, write that on your label, along with "Elderberry Syrup" and the date. Cool and funnel into bottles. Keep in the fridge for up to 2 weeks.

This recipe produces 35 doses. To get one dose, divide the total amount you have by 35. In general, adults can take 1 tablespoon every 3-4 hours (up to six times a day) if they're sick, while kids over 1 should take 1 teaspoon per dose.

17. Sage-Infused Honey

Used for:

Sore throat.

Sage and honey are both great for treating a sore throat. Sage is astringent, anti-bacterial, and anti-inflammatory. Raw honey also contains powerful medicinal components and coats the throat. Together, they form a tasty and strong cough syrup. Because this syrup is just sage and honey, it can also be used in culinary recipes if you want!

Ingredients:

- 1 cup raw honey
- 1 cup sage leaves, fresh

Directions:

1. Wash and dry sage. Trim leaves off stems if you haven't already. Put the sage into your glass jar, filling up to ¾ of the way full.

2. Pour honey into the jar. If it moves really slowly, you can heat it a little in a double boiler, but do it very gently and only until it's just becoming smoother.

3. Heat kills many of the raw honey's medicinal properties. When honey is in your jar, stir. Seal and label the jar. Let the honey infuse for at least a week before using, stirring once a day.

4. Store in a cool, dry, and dark place. It will be at its best for 1 year. When spooning out honey, always use a clean spoon to avoid contamination.

18. Ginger-Thyme Cough Drops

Used for:

Sore throat.

Homemade cough drops are tasty and a great vehicle for your herbs. They're also a great gift around cold and flu season. Ginger is an anti-inflammatory while thyme has been used as a sore throat and coughing remedy for years.

Ingredients:

- 3-5 slices ginger, fresh (or 1 teaspoon ground ginger)
- ½ cup thyme, fresh (or 3 tablespoons thyme, dried)
- 1 cup water
- 1 tablespoon lemon juice
- 1 cup raw white sugar
- 1 tablespoon honey

Directions:

1. Line two baking trays with baking paper. In a saucepot, bring your water to a boil. Add the ginger and thyme. Reduce the heat to a simmer and steep for 10 minutes. Strain and set aside for now.

2. To make the sugar syrup, put the sugar, lemon juice, and ⅓ cup + 1 ½ tablespoons of the herb-infused water in a pot. Turn on the heat. Stir constantly as the sugar dissolves. It should take about 7-10 minutes. Once the sugar is dissolved, reduce the heat and cook for another 7-10 minutes. When the mixture hits 300-degrees (use a candy thermometer), it's ready.

3. Drop cough drop-sized dots of the syrup on your baking sheets and cool. When they're hard, move to a labeled container. Use within 4 weeks.

19. Chickweed Tincture

Used for:

Skin irritations, acne, scrapes, bumps, bruises.

This tincture can be applied to irritated skin, acne, scrapes, and any other area where you need skin healing. A standard dose (20-75 drops) can also be added to tea for digestive issues like constipation.

Ingredients:

- ¾ cup chickweed, fresh, chopped
- 1 cup 80/100 proof alcohol (like vodka)

Directions:

1. Put your chickweed in a clean jar. Pour vodka over the herbs, so they're completely covered. Seal and label the jar. Store the jar in a cool, dark, and dry place for 4-8 weeks. Every few days, shake well.
2. When the steeping time is up, line a sieve with cheesecloth and strain the tincture. Funnel into a

dark-colored glass dropper bottle. Label the jar and keep it out of direct sunlight. The tincture should last up to five years.

20. Parsley Tea

Used for:

Indigestion, kidney health, bladder health, cramping.

Parsley is full of antioxidants and vitamins. It's anti-inflammatory and has been used to ease period cramps. If you have kidney disease, high blood pressure, or diabetes, talk to your doctor before drinking parsley tea. If you're pregnant, don't drink the tea. No one should drink it longer than two weeks in a row.

Ingredients (makes 2 cups tea):

- 4 tablespoons parsley, fresh, chopped (or 4 teaspoons parsley, dried)
- 2 cups hot water
- Raw honey to taste

Directions:

1. Steep parsley in hot water for 5-7 minutes. You can use a tea strainer or steep the leaves right in the water and strain later.
2. Add raw honey for sweetness. Lemon juice is also tasty.

21. Valerian Root Capsules

Used for:

Insomnia, headaches, stomach aches.

Valerian is a powerful medicinal herb with its benefits found in the root. People who don't want to use sleeping pills often turn to valerian root instead. It also eases headaches and stomach aches. It should not be used if you're on anti-anxiety medication.

Ingredients:

- 3000-6000 mg valerian root, dried
- 10 capsules

Directions:

1. To powder your valerian, use a mortar and pestle, or a food processor. Grind until you get a sandy texture. Fill the capsules. If you're using a machine, you'll pour the powdered herb over the machine base into one-half of the capsules. Spread the powder over the

capsules to fill them. With the tamper, press the powder down, so it's packed into the capsules. Keep spreading with the card and tampering until the capsules are full.

2. Sweep off any extra powder. Go ahead and take the bottom off the stand. Put the top of the capsule machine on the base and press down. The capsules should be packed now. Over a container, press down on the back of the machine's top part to release the capsules. That's it!

Based on research for capsules, we saw that herbalists often recommend shaking a little bit of valerian powder around in the container, so you'll taste a little of the root when you take a capsule. Tasting it helps your body recognize what it's consuming, which can help it respond better to the powder.

CONCLUSION

Nature, of course, has not always been regarded with apprehension. Much as when they were angry, the spirits of animals and other facets of nature could be dangerous, but they might also be beneficial when they were happy. For one, the Native Americans believed that herbs and even animals' organs were full of enormous healing powers. During their various curing rituals, they also called on the spirits of animals for help. It was believed that various species had special characteristics and qualities, such as cunning, intellect, and courage. During healing rituals, Native Americans may call for individual animal spirits, asking each in return to share their special gifts with the person being healed. Still, of course, doctors are unlikely to consider calling on the spirits of eagles and bears to regulate blood pressure or cure arthritis but depending on how it is handled, they are very mindful of nature's ability to cure or hurt

Native American medicine addresses the healing of the whole person, and therefore uses the holistic approach to healing and cure. We know that health requires some kind of balance. These days we come across medical problems like some types of cancer, which defy all types of treatments. Yet, when natural remedies are taken, and the environment is taken care of, the water, the air we breathe, and the food we eat, all of these bring some kind of balance in every sphere of life, not just the physical.

Many medical problems can be resolved by changing our lifestyle and the social connections we have with those around us. We can reduce stress and depression by caring for others who also care about us so that we can find inward peace. Emotional imbalance is as much a problem as physical illnesses and diseases. We need to deal with our emotions to be able to embrace holistic healing and cure.

With this book on your shelf, you will always have the ancient wisdom of Native Americans at your fingertips. Remember to investigate every substance you take and don't delegate responsibility for your healing to anyone but experts.

Thank you for reading. Stay healthy!

CPSIA information can be obtained
at www.ICGtesting.com
Printed in the USA
BVHW041506180321
602887BV00012B/1719

9 781914 373282